THE
WHIPLASH
BOOK

*How you can deal with
a whiplash injury –
based on the latest
medical research*

London: The Stationery Office

Help and advice from colleagues too
numerous to mention is gratefully acknowledged.

© The Stationery Office 2001

Applications for reproduction should be made in writing to The
Stationery Office Limited, St Crispins, Duke Street, Norwich NR3
1PD.

The information in this book is intended solely for the purpose of
providing general information; it is not intended to be, nor is it to be
treated as, a substitute for professional medical advice. Always seek
the advice of your doctor for any questions you may have regarding
a medical condition.

A CIP catalogue record for this book is available from the British
Library.

A Library of Congress CIP catalogue record has been applied for.

WHY THE WHIPLASH BOOK?

This booklet gives you the best and most up-to-date advice on how to deal with whiplash, recover quickly and avoid long term pain and disability. It is based on the latest research. Even if you have never had a whiplash injury, you may want to read it and keep it handy.

Neck pain is very common, even without an accident or injury. With busy roads, about 1 in 200 people now have a minor neck injury or whiplash each year. But fortunately, serious or permanent damage is rare.

We have now learned a great deal about whiplash but people are still confused and get conflicting advice about the best way to tackle it. This booklet sets out the facts and shows you how you can get better quickly. How you react and what you do yourself is usually more important than the exact nature of the injury or the treatment you receive.

A car accident is certainly disturbing and frightening. Even a minor whiplash can be very painful, and it's natural to think that something dreadful might have happened to you. But stop and look at the facts:

WHIPLASH FACTS

- Permanent damage is rare. The long-term outlook is good.
- Most whiplash injuries are not serious. There is usually no damage to the bones, discs or nerves in the spine. Serious injuries are nearly always detected early.
- Some people only develop pain a day or two after the accident. That is a good sign. It means the damage to your neck is not serious.
- Everyone knows that whiplash causes neck pain, but some people also get low back pain. Again, there is rarely any serious damage to the back.
- It is not uncommon to get headaches after whiplash from tension in the neck. Some people get other symptoms such as arm or jaw pain, or dizziness. All these usually get better along with the neck pain. The advice in this booklet talks mainly about neck pain, but you should find it helpful for these other symptoms too.
- The acute pain usually improves within days or a few weeks, at least enough to get on with your life.

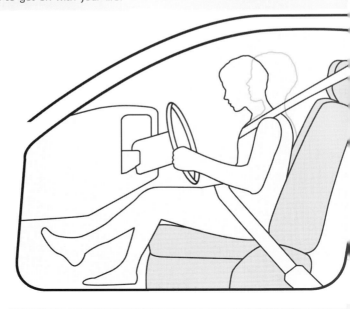

- Sometimes aches and pains can persist or recur for quite a long time after a whiplash injury. But that still does not mean it is serious. Even if pain does continue it need not become unbearable or disabling. The pain usually settles eventually - though it can certainly be frustrating that no one can predict exactly when! Yet most people can get going quite quickly, even while they still have some symptoms.

- What you do in the early stages is very important. Rest for more than a day or two usually does not help and may actually prolong pain and disability.

- Your neck is designed for movement – a lot of movement. The sooner you get your neck moving and doing your ordinary activities as normally as possible, the sooner you will feel better.

- The people who cope best with whiplash are those who stay active, exercise their neck, and get on with life despite the pain.

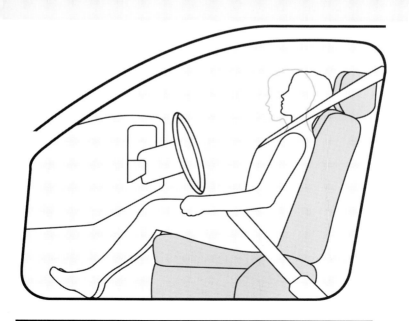

THE ANATOMY OF WHIPLASH

Your spine, and that includes your neck as well as your
back, is one of the strongest parts of your body. It is
made of solid bony blocks joined by discs to give it
strength and flexibility. It is reinforced by strong ligaments.
It is surrounded by large and powerful muscles that
protect it. It is surprisingly difficult to do any serious
damage to your neck. Most everyday traffic shunts are
not violent enough to cause lasting damage.

Despite what you may have heard:

• Whiplash injuries usually affect just the working parts of
  your neck – the muscles and ligaments and small joints.
  These have a natural ability to repair and restore
  themselves.
• Some people get shooting pains or tingling in their
  arms, but whiplash injuries rarely cause a slipped disc
  or a trapped nerve. Minor nerve irritation like this
  usually gets better by itself. Whiplash injuries hardly
  ever need surgery.
• X-rays and MRI scans can detect serious spinal injuries,
  but they usually do not help in an ordinary whiplash.
  They may even be misleading because most of what
  they show in your neck has nothing to do with the injury.
  Doctors sometimes call these 'degenerative changes'
  which is a rather alarming technical term, but that is
  not damage or arthritis. These are the normal changes
  with age – just like grey hair.

Often your doctor or therapist cannot pinpoint the source
of the pain. It is frustrating not to know exactly what is
wrong. But in another way that is good news. It confirms
that you don't have any serious damage in your neck.

After a whiplash injury your neck is simply not moving properly and working as it should. You may think of the injury as causing your neck to seize up. So what you need to do is get it moving.

Warning Signs

If you have a violent accident and your neck is very painful you should go to Accident & Emergency or see your doctor, just to make sure there is no serious damage. That is particularly important if you have:

> Been unconscious.
> Disturbed vision.
> Severe muscle spasm, or your neck is in an abnormal posture.
> Pins and needles, numbness or weakness in your arms or legs.
> Any difficulty with balance or walking.

Don't let that list worry you too much. Fortunately, serious damage to the spine is rare and can usually be excluded quickly and with confidence.

THE NEW APPROACH

The old fashioned treatment for whiplash was rest and immobilisation.
Some people with back or neck pain went to bed or used a collar for
months on end, just waiting for the pain to disappear. But rest is the worst
possible treatment, because in the long term it actually prolongs the pain:
> You get stiff.

> Your muscles get weak.

> You lose physical fitness.

> You get depressed.

> The pain feels worse.

> It is harder and harder to get going again.

No wonder it didn't work! The message is now clear: PROLONGED
INACTIVITY IS BAD FOR WHIPLASH.

Of course you might be limited in how much you can do for the first few
days if the pain is severe. But only for a few days. And don't think of that
as a treatment, but rather look on these limitations as a short-term and
undesirable consequence of the injury. The most important thing is to get
moving and get active again as soon as you can.

MOVEMENT IS GOOD FOR YOU – AND FOR WHIPLASH

Your whole body must stay active to stay healthy. It thrives on use. USE IT
OR LOSE IT.

Regular physical activity:
> Gives you strong bones.

> Develops fit active muscles.

> Keeps you supple.

> Makes you fit.

> Makes you feel good.

> Releases natural chemicals that reduce the pain.

Even when you are sore, you can make a start without putting too much stress on your neck. There are many forms of exercise that can help whiplash. Some examples are:

> Simple neck exercises.

> Any form of aerobic exercises.

> Keep fit exercises.

> Yoga.

> Walking.

> Most daily activities and many hobbies.

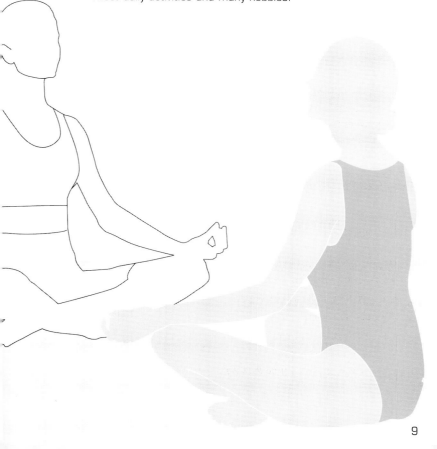

Different exercises suit different people and you must find for yourself what best suits you and your neck. Rearrange your life to get regular physical activity at some time every day. Do something you enjoy, because then you will keep it up. The important thing is not which exercise you chose, but that you keep mobile and maintain regular activity even if it's a bit uncomfortable at first.

The faster you get back to normal activities and get on with your life the better, even if you still have some pain. Using stiff joints and muscles and making them work again often does hurt at first. Athletes accept that when they start training their muscles can hurt and they have to work through a pain barrier. But that does not mean they are doing any damage. The same is true for whiplash.

Pain killers and other treatments can help to control the pain to let you get started, but you still have to work through the pain. There is no other way. You have a straight choice: rest and deteriorate or get active and recover.

Do not fall into the trap of thinking it will be easier to get active in a week or two, next month, next year. It won't! The chances are that the longer you put it off, the harder it will be to get going again.

HOW TO DEAL WITH A WHIPLASH INJURY.

Whiplash injuries can be very painful, even if there is little to see. However, because there's no serious damage, you can:

> Use something to control the pain.
> Do neck exercises – some good ones are shown in the following pages
> Stay active and get on with your life.
> Modify your activities for a time, if necessary.

You will have good days and bad days. That's normal, and it's part of getting better.

Control of Pain

There are some treatments that can help. They may not remove the pain completely, but they should control it enough to let you get moving and active. They do not cure your injury. Your body does that – with your help.

Pain killers
You can use pain killers to help manage your pain and you should not hesitate if you need them. Paracetamol is the simplest and safest pain killer. Or you can use anti-inflammatory tablets like Ibuprofen. It may surprise you, but these are often the most effective for neck and back pains if you take them regularly every 4-6 hours.

You should usually take the pain killers for a few days, but you may need to take them for a week or two. Take them regularly and do not wait till your pain is out of control. Do not take Ibuprofen or Aspirin if you are pregnant or if you have asthma, indigestion or an ulcer.

Collars
A collar is sometimes given for immediate support and relief, but research now shows that after the first few days it may delay recovery. So the faster you can do without the collar and get your neck moving again the better.

Heat & cold
Local heat or cold can be used for short-term relief of pain and to relax muscle spasm. In the first 48 hours you can try a cold pack on the sore area for 5-10 minutes at a time - a bag of frozen peas wrapped in a damp towel. Other people prefer heat - a hot water bottle, a bath or a shower.

Manipulation
Most doctors now agree that manipulation or mobilisation can help. This is safe if done by a qualified professional: osteopaths, chiropractors, some physiotherapists and a few doctors with special training. It is probably most effective in the early stages, especially if you combine it with getting active. You should begin to feel the benefit within a few sessions and there is no value in treatment for months on end.

Traction
Traction is sometimes used for short-term pain relief but it does not have any long-term effect. Its only value is if it helps you to start getting active.

Other Treatments

Many other treatments such as massage, electro-therapy machines, acupuncture or alternative medicine are used for neck pain and some people feel they help. It is up to you to find what helps to ease your symptoms. But be realistic. Despite the claims, these treatments rarely provide a magic answer. Once again, you should feel any benefit quite quickly and there is no value in treatment for months on end. What really matters is whether they help you get mobile and active and so get yourself better.

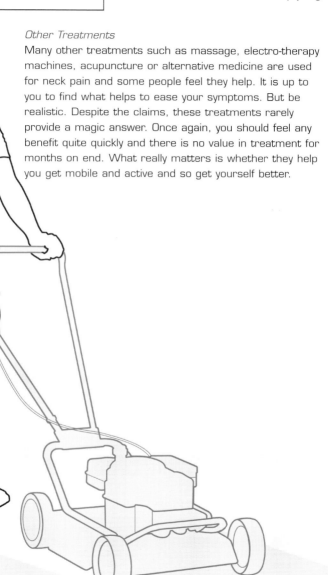

Neck exercises

Exercise is good for whiplash and it's a way to treat yourself. Simple neck exercises are safe and effective. They reduce the pain and help you get on with your life. They get your neck moving again by stretching tight muscles and joints, and prevent the working parts from seizing up. Don't worry if they make you a bit sore to start with – that is usually a sign you are actually making progress! It's the improvement in function that's important, because once you get full movement and are back to full activity the pain should ease off.

There is no single exercise that is right for everyone. So don't be afraid to experiment to find what works best for you and your neck. In general terms, you should progressively stretch your neck in all directions. You should move to the point of pain, then gradually try to go a little bit further each session.

To give you an idea of the sort of exercises you can do yourself, here are some suggestions to get you started. Obviously you need to exercise your neck, but it also helps to work your shoulders. You can exercise sitting or standing, or if that's too painful you could try some of them lying on your back. Or you could make a start in a warm bath or shower. If your pain seems worse, do them less frequently and through a smaller range rather than stop altogether.

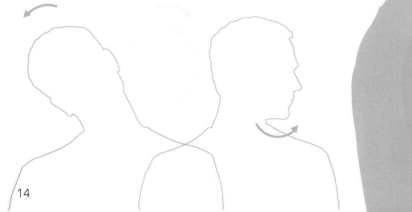

Then as the pain eases you can build up again. If a particular exercise makes you dizzy you should try a different one. You should avoid rolling your head round.

Neck stretching
You need to go in all directions – forwards and backwards, leaning over to both sides and turning your head right and left. Move your head slowly in one direction then in the opposite direction as far as you feel you can. Repeat about ten times in each direction every hour or so.

Shoulder stretching
Moving your arms stretches your shoulder muscles –
> Shrug your shoulders while breathing in and then relax them whilst breathing out. Try rolling them at the same time.
> Circle your arms, one at a time, backwards and forwards – like swimming crawl and backstroke. Bend the elbows if that's easier.

Repeat about ten times in each direction every hour or so.

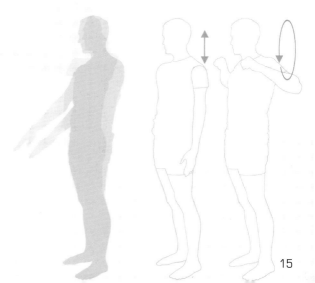

You should also do some strengthening and coordination exercises. Strengthening exercises will reduce both fatigue and pain. Coordination exercises improve the control of neck movements. These exercises help you get safely back to normal activity.

Neck strengthening
The idea is to make your neck muscles work without actually moving your head. Put your hand on the side of your head and apply increasing pressure. As you resist, you will feel your muscles contracting. Maintain the force for 10 seconds and then gradually release. Repeat to the other side. Similarly, push forwards against both hands on your forehead, and then backwards against your clasped hands behind your head.

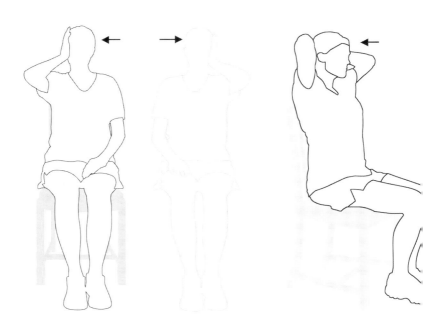

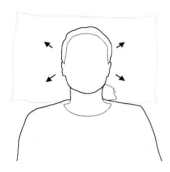

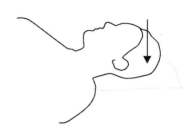

Neck coordination

Lie on your back with your head on a thin pillow. Push your head backwards into the centre of the pillow. Whilst still pressing down and looking straight up, push towards each corner of the pillow in turn, without really moving your head. This helps you learn to control your neck muscles and movements.

If you need extra help you could see a physiotherapist, who is an expert on exercise and rehabilitation. But physiotherapists can't do the exercises for you. They may show you how and help you to get started, but you have to put in the effort and do the work yourself. So the sooner you are doing the exercises yourself the better. And once again there's no value in going for treatment for months on end.

Anxiety, stress and muscle tension

Anxiety and stress can increase the amount of pain we feel. Tension can cause muscle spasm and the muscles themselves can become painful.

It is normal to be anxious after a whiplash injury, especially if it's not getting better as fast as you would like. You may get conflicting advice – even from doctors and therapists, or from your family and friends – which may make you uncertain of what best to do. Trust the advice in this booklet – it comes from the latest research. Remember, serious damage is rare and the long-term outlook is good. So do not let fear and worry hold back your recovery.

Stress can also aggravate or prolong pain. If stress is a problem you need to recognise it at an early stage and try to do something about it. You cannot always avoid stress, but it is possible to learn to reduce its effects by controlled breathing, muscle relaxation and mental calming techniques. Exercise is also an excellent way of reducing stress and tension.

Muscle relaxation
Lie comfortably on your back, knees bent up, in a quiet room.
The idea is to contract a set of muscles and then let them go – simply spending a few minutes doing this for various parts of the body will ease any muscle tension and reduce stress.

Controlled breathing

Lie comfortably on your back with eyes closed and knees bent up over a pillow.

Breath in slowly through the nose and feel your abdomen rise – breath out through your mouth and feel your abdomen gently fall.

Try this for a few minutes – some people fall asleep!

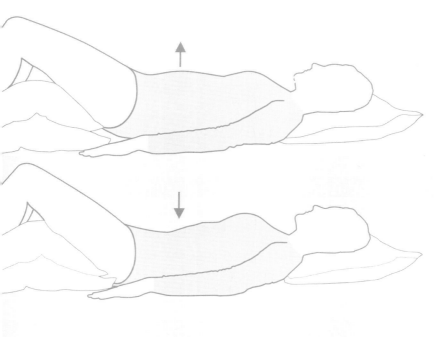

The risk of chronic pain

There has been a lot of research in recent years to identify people at risk of developing long term pain and disability. What may surprise you is that most of the warning signs are about what we feel and do rather than medical findings.

Early warning signs of people at risk:
> Belief that you have a serious injury or damage. Unable to accept reassurance.
> Belief that hurt means harm and that you will become disabled.
> Avoiding movement or activity due to fear of doing damage.
> Continued rest and avoiding normal daily activities instead of getting on with your life.
> Waiting for someone to fix it rather than believing that you can help yourself recover.
> Unable to see any improvement at all after 1 or 2 weeks.
> Becoming withdrawn and depressed.

It may be difficult to stop yourself reacting like this. Some people around you may become unsympathetic if your symptoms do not settle quickly, but that's not your fault. The situation develops gradually and you may not even notice. But that is why it is so important to get going as soon as possible *before* you develop chronic pain. If you – or your family and friends – do spot some of these early warning signs, you need to do something about it. Now, before it's too late. Stop and think about what is happening to you and where you are going. Use the advice in this booklet to work out what you can do to change direction and get on with your life. If you need extra help to get going, you should ask your doctor or therapist.

You may meet a practical problem here. Doctors and therapists deal best with clear-cut diseases and injuries for which they have a cure. Our health services are not so good at dealing with more ordinary symptoms like neck pain or whiplash. For example, it's no good staying off work and doing nothing for weeks on end to attend therapy. Or waiting months to see a surgeon who will just tell you that you do not need an operation. That simply delays your recovery! Which is why it really does depend on what you do yourself. You also have to make it clear to your doctor or therapist that you realise all this and what you really want is help to get on with your life.

If you are still off work after 3-6 weeks, you are at risk of developing long-term problems. There is a 10% risk you will still be off work in a year's time. You could even lose your job. Before you get to that stage you really must face up to the problem and take urgent action.

How to stay active

If your pain is severe you may have to rest for a few days or even stay off work. But as we've explained, too much rest is bad for you and the sooner you start getting mobile and active again the better.

Fortunately, you do not need a fully mobile neck to do most of the things you want to do. You can do most daily activities if you think about them first or change the way you do them.

The idea is to strike a balance between being as active as you can and not putting too much strain on your neck. The basic rules are simple: *Keep moving. Do not stay in one position for too long. Move about before you stiffen up. Move a little further and faster every day. Don't completely avoid things, just alter the way you do them.*

Sitting Chose a chair and position that is comfortable for you – experiment. Get up and stretch regularly – take advantage of TV adverts!

Desk work Adjust the height of your chair to suit your desk. Adjust your keyboard and VDU so that your neck and shoulders are comfortable. Keep the mouse close. Get up and stretch regularly.

Driving Adjust your seat so that you can hold the steering wheel comfortably. Stop regularly for a few minutes break. Get out of the car, walk about and stretch. Make sure your headrest is level with the top of your head and no more than two inches behind it.

Carrying and shopping Think if you need to carry it all. Carry things hugged to your body or split the load between both hands. Use a trolley.

Daily activities and hobbies Do each activity for a short period. Keep changing activities. Use your arms at or below shoulder level.

Sports Continuing with your normal sports is fine if it's non-impact or non-contact. Reduce intensity e.g. walking or cycling instead of running or rugby. Swimming - try a different stroke – back stroke, side stroke, crawl.

Sleeping Find what pillow is most comfortable for you – higher or lower, softer or firmer. Experiment. Take painkillers an hour before you go to bed.

Getting on with your life

It's important to maintain the momentum of your life. Doing things will distract you from the pain, and your neck will not get any worse at work than it will at home. It is important to remain at work if you possibly can. If you can't, it helps to get back to work as soon as possible, even if you still have some pain. The longer you are inactive and off work the more likely you are to develop long term pain and disability.

If you are seeing a doctor or therapist, tell them about your work. You may also want to discuss the problem with your supervisor or employer. Tell them about any parts of your job that may be difficult for you to begin with, but stress that you want to be at work. Offer suggestions about how to overcome these problems. You might even show them this booklet.

Most people can manage to get back to most normal activities quite quickly – usually within days or a couple of weeks. If not, you should be taking more positive action or getting help to become fully active.

If you are not back to work within about a month you should be talking to your doctor, your therapist and your employer about how and when you will. Your occupational health department or health and safety rep may be able to assist. Temporary modification to your job or pattern of work may help at this stage.

What doctors can and can't do

Doctors can diagnose and treat the few serious spinal injuries, but they have no quick fix for whiplash. So you must be realistic about what you can expect from doctors and therapists. Even though serious damage is very rare, you may still feel the need to check and that is quite reasonable.

Your doctor can:

> Make sure you don't have any serious damage and reassure you.
> Suggest various treatments to help control your pain.
> Advise you on how you can best deal with the pain and get on with your life.

The main thing is to accept that reassurance and don't let needless worry delay your recovery. You must share responsibility for your own progress. Even today, some doctors and therapists may be a little hesitant about letting you take control of things. You may have to ask straight out to let them know this really is what you want to do.

IT'S YOUR NECK

We have shown you that whiplash is usually not a serious injury and it should not disable you unless you let it. You've got the facts and the most up-to-date advice about how to deal with it. The important thing now is to get on with your life. How your neck affects you depends on how you react to the pain and what you do about it yourself.

There is no instant answer. You will have the normal ups and downs for a while. But think of it this way:

There are two types of sufferer:

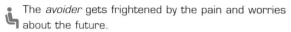

One who *avoids* activity

and one who *copes*

The *avoider* gets frightened by the pain and worries about the future.

- The *avoider* is afraid that hurting always means further damage - it doesn't.
- The *avoider* rests a lot, withdraws from life and just waits for the pain to get better.

The *coper* knows that the pain will get better and does not fear the future.

- The *coper* carries on as normally as possible.
- The *coper* deals with the pain by being positive, staying active and getting on with life.

Who suffers most?

 Avoiders suffer most. They have pain for longer, they have more time off work and they can become disabled.

 Copers get better faster, enjoy life more and have less trouble in the long run.

So how do I become a Coper and prevent unnecessary suffering?

Follow these guidelines – you really can help yourself.

Live life as normally as possible. This is much better than giving in to the pain.

• Keep up daily activities – they will not cause damage. Within reason, the more active you are the better.

• Start gradually and do a little more each day so you can see the progress you are making.

• Get on with your life and either stay at work or go back to work as soon as possible. If necessary, ask if you can get lighter or modified duties for a week or two.

• Be patient. It's normal to get aches or twinges for a time.

• Don't rely on painkillers alone. Stay positive and take control of the pain yourself.

• Don't stay at home or give up doing things you enjoy.

• Don't get frightened. Continuing pain does not mean you are going to become an invalid.

• Don't get gloomy on the down days.

27

Remember:

- Whiplash injuries are common but they rarely cause any serious damage.

- Even when it is very painful that usually doesn't mean there's any serious damage to your neck. Hurt is not the same as harm.

- Rest for more than a day or two is usually bad for you.

- Keeping moving and staying active will help you get better faster.

- The sooner you get going, the sooner you will get better.

- If you don't manage to get back to most normal activities quite quickly, you should seek additional help.

- You have to get on with your life. Don't let a whiplash injury take over.

Printed in the United Kingdom by The Stationery Office Ltd, London
TJ5598 C30 11/01 669283 19585